YOGA LIFE SAVERS

My Yoga Story Handbook.

Holly Kirkpatrick Ulrich

Eva Marie Originals

ISBN-13: 9781234567890
ISBN-10: 1477123456

Cover design by: Art Painter
Library of Congress Control Number: 2018675309
Printed in the United States of America

CONTENTS

INTRODUCTION

When I was a young girl, I read everything I could get my hands on. Growing up in a north western Canada boom and bust industry town in the 1980's, I loved to read. Not only was it something to *do* in our small town - with reading, I had freedom. I was allowed to choose whatever I wanted to read. I guessed this was because my parent's valued education, and literacy, and having this choice encouraged me to read. I was allowed to be led by my curiosity, and so I read.

At one point I stumbled across a small paperback simply called Yoga. I don't remember who wrote it. but I remember the author explaining how she practiced headstands even if she was on an airplane! Since then, I have read many more books on yoga and everything to do with it. But I have also thought about the woman who wrote that book so long ago and how because she wrote it, my life was influenced in a small yet profound way.

I've also thought about the many opportunities that have come my way over the years. Yoga training, and inspirational teachers and moments, too numerous to even count . I have always felt a deep gratitude for my good fortune.

After finishing art school, it just so happened I was able to concentrate and dedicate a few years of my life full time to yoga. This was at the turn of the millennium. I always found this so profound considering Yoga is such an ancient scientific system for all aspects of health- Physical, Mental, and Spiritual.

So much is going on in the world and so much has happened

and is happening all the time. The Beautiful thing is no matter who or where you are or what is going on around you, you can always practice yoga. Why? Because it takes very little set up, and everyone always feels better after practicing Yoga, and feeling better makes the world better. Yoga essentially means Yolk- it helps us to center ourselves and feel our connection to the universe and all things.

With all that I have learned, so many mixed emotions rise up about being able to share some of it with you now. First and foremost I feel strongly that now is the time. I need to get this information out into the world right now, without a moment to spare. To share with you some simple yet valuable and powerful techniques and information that could essentially save your life! Or at the very least help your life quality or that of someone near you. I have internalized and practiced to the point that it is inside me, that it might help assist you along your journey as I have found it has helped me.

I wonder at how long it has taken me to get to this point. The processing, reflection and reviewing, and then coming back to the gift. This is about now and the gift of the present, so here it is. For you as you are, in this moment, and with awareness of the breath that animates your life.

With Much Love,
Holly

PS - Be advised:
The information contained here is from what I have found helpful over many years. I welcome and encourage you to find what works best for you. You are welcome to do things differently. The information contained in these pages are what I have come back to again and again and what works for me.
It's a crazy world we live in, things are moving fast. When things get crazy or even when things are going along on an even keel for you, and when things are great? How do you hold it

together how do you integrate? What do you honestly turn to? How do you stay present and enjoy the fullness of everything our lives have to offer us? How do you work things out and get through the challenges? How do you quiet your busy mind?

This little book has been incubating in me for a long time, thanks to many great yoga teachers and my own practice . I hope you will find some suggestions that resonate with you to use right now - to transform challenges and difficulties into opportunities. This starts by embracing and accepting who you are right now, and staying with yourself with your center core into the next moment and the next. The time has come to share. I have wondered when it would happen, staying as present as possible along the way and the time is now!

Please remember!
This is about being curious and letting yourself be where you are at and gently exploring the edges of your abilities. It is absolutely completely NOT about wrenching your body into strange positions. Go slow and easy like the tortoise who won the race.
It is also, of course, not a substitute for going to see a doctor.
If something does not feel right for you, always listen carefully to your own inner voice.

Everything I say is a suggestion. Please take what works for you and leave the rest. And on that note, I would suggest you may like to visualize yourself going through the motions as you read through the book, picturing yourself moving in and out of the yoga poses, so as to be more able to remember the subtle instructions when you actually get to trying them out on your mat.

May you enjoy reading this book and learn as much as I did creating it. May you be enriched and discover the simple joy of yoga.

1. HELPFUL EQUIPMENT

One of the beautiful things about yoga is you don't need much.

What You Will Need To Practice Yoga: Think Minimalist

The main thing is to clear away distractions.
These wise words of wisdom have I contemplated in my life!

- Clear-Away-Distractions
- A Yoga Mat

It's nice to have a yoga mat, aka "sticky mat" for practicing yoga.

It gives you a grippy surface so you won't slip around. Yoga mats also give us an important edge to align our bodies with to help us be aware of our own body in relation to our surroundings. Think of the mat edges almost like four straight edge rulers you work within.

Thinking back, I spent a long time borrowing a mat in the class I took before I was ready to commit to buying one. These days yoga classes expect you to provide your own. They sell them everywhere these days. Spray your new yoga mat down in the shower with hot water to wash off any slippery film, then hang to dry.

No Yoga mat? No problem! You can practice without. I can assure you I practice yoga all the time as I go through my daily life. But a mat really is a good investment.

- A Cozy Blanket, or Three!
Have a blanket to cover up with to stay warm, to hide under, for comfort and yes for security. If there is one thing important for us to own at all, I would say, it is a blanket. Blankets are the best! In yoga they can be used to prop us up, or support us. But mainly to stay warm in the resting position of Savasana. Any blanket will do. Cotton woven blankets as found from Mexico work really well. I have a fuzzy fleecy one I like to use lately.

- An Eye Pillow-
These are amazing and not to be underestimated- I have owned a couple. A little pillow filled with flax seeds and lavender. They have ones with sand in them too, (Sand bag weights are also used in another form of restorative yoga practice) I actually don't have an eye pillow right now- and life goes on. I am using one of my son's muslin baby blankets to cover my eyes in Savasana, and it works great too. A Silky scarf would also work well.

- Clothing -Comfortable clothes that aren't too loose or baggy.

   We are always looking for the 'just right' factor here, always in practicing yoga. Clothing to practice in is no exception. This will vary a little from person to person. I notice I often am wearing my regular day to day clothes when I fit in a practice. Otherwise, I look for a top that doesn't bag out, droop open or fall forward if I bend over, and pants or shorts that are snug but stretchy. Also, important comfortable underwear, it doesn't have to be a sports bra, maybe you need a bra, maybe you don't even need a shirt. The main thing is snug well-fitting clothing. You can wear a looser top over if you wish and be able to take it off when necessary. Layers are always good, right?

- Wall Space- It may seem crazy but it's funny how often I notice wall space lacking. We fill our homes covering almost every surface. If you can dedicate a wall to yoga practice it's a wonderful thing. The space needs to be as tall as you are, as wide as you are tall and go out as tall as you are.

- Also Quiet- Ideally a bit of time where you won't be distracted.
- I used to take this for granted - You need to have quiet- turn off phones- lock the door to your room or office- Ask the people around you to give you this space- This is more challenging than it might seem- but over time you can carve it out for yourself and train the people around you to respect it.

Once you have these simple things taken care of it will also help to eliminate many distractions.

Additional Equipment

You may also acquire the following helpful items. You can get by with most of the items I have mentioned, but it is really a nice gift to yourself to have these things if and when you can. Or find a yoga studio that uses these props. If you phone around to classes you could ask if they use props? Props can be very helpful regardless of your level of experience.

- Yoga block - a firm block usually made of foam or cork. You sit on these and it makes sitting on the ground easier for many people. Including me- For instance, it might sound silly but I had one around while my son was a toddler, and I could play with him on the floor for way longer when I could prop myself up under my sit bones with the block, you'd be surprised.

- Yoga strap - a long strap with a belt loop. It can help you extend further into poses. Eg: take a strap and reach up- drop it down your back, now reach around and grab the strap as high up as you can comfortably reach- And Voila! No need to reach your hands together behind your back and you still get a wonderful stretch.
- Bolster- This is a big firm cylindrical pillow. These are so nice to have, I have felt everyone should have one, to the point that I have gifted them to family members. They are great for sitting on, laying over top of, and propping up your hips.

Why Do We Need Props?

All the props do is help make your experience of yoga more comfortable and help open up the tightness in your body.

Like I said at the beginning of this chapter, you really don't need much, you can even get away without a yoga mat for a while. It's really about your connection to the earth, your awareness of yourself in space, and accepting yourself exactly where you're at. If you go to do a pose and you find your hands or feet are slipping, you will see why a yoga mat can be helpful. Coming back to your center as I will also be speaking about, will allow you to practice the poses and accept to what extent that you can in the moment. With a little creativity and imagination you can even practice variations of many poses simplified sitting in a chair. The reality is you will be reading this before trying any of it, so I would recommend as you read, you visualize yourself trying things. Picturing yourself in the poses in your mind's eye, is a powerful exercise in itself.

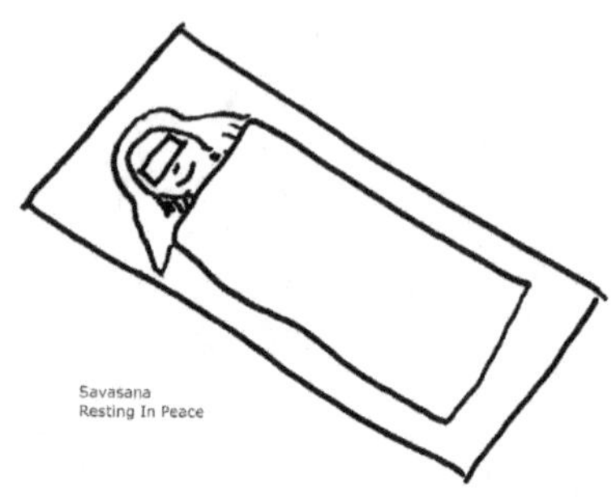

2.
BEGIN WITH THE END IN MIND

Savasana- Shah-vah-sah-nah

Rest In Peace. Corpse Pose. Deep Full Body Relaxation.

Also sometimes referred to (by me) as –"The 12-Minute Break"

Begin with the End in Mind.

When I was in high school, I had a Drama teacher who always referred to the morning break as the "12-minute break". Because you guessed it - it was 12 minutes long!

It was one of the times in the day, when we didn't have to be in class, and although we had to navigate what was going on around us socially in the hall and with schoolmates, we had the option where we didn't have to do or think about anything- just like in Savasana.

I was fortunate to be first introduced to this wonderful delicious pose once on a drama trip with the same Drama teacher at a Provincial Arts Festival- We went to a Farm Based Theater where we played with masks and the leader of the workshop also led us through a guided deep relaxation. We all piled into a barn, filled with hay bales. Being guided, it was actually more like Savasana in combination with Yoga Nidra, which is very similar and I explain towards the end of the book. In any case, it might sound funny, but I honestly remember feeling that experience, in that moment changed my life. That somehow this was very important for me to learn, to practice, and to learn to share with others.There is so many other places in our lives where it is demanded we be productive and be thinking, our society highly values the rational and logical, in savasana, I found a place where I could practice being and it was like a precious gift.

I have always remembered this experience and want to share it now to help you understand how important it really is.

For my own Savasana – the Do Nothing Pose- 12 minutes actually works quite nicely. IN my opinion the best yoga classes hold space for at least 10 minutes of this pose at the end of the class. I like 20 minutes to really go deeper. But 12 minutes will work with a little bit of practice and most people can spare 12 minutes, right?!

Savasana allows you to absorb the benefits of your full yoga practice and let go of anything you no longer need. Lying completely still dissolves tension.

Thinking takes more energy than any physical activity so this is not a time to go over your schedule for the week. The idea is to completely relax your whole body, every muscle, every bone, all our internal organs, and most challenging to relax and rest our minds. By doing this tension begins to dissipate. Notice the areas holding onto tension in your body as you do this, just scan through, and give those areas permission to let go. Those little areas are just waiting for your instruction for the whisper to,"let go."

*Set your timer 10-20 minutes and lay completely still under a blanket. A small light blanket, eye pillow or scarf draped over the eyes is helpful too.

Be in a place you won't be disturbed- This is something I took for granted over the many years when I did not have a child. If you have children- you may need to do this when they are in bed or not around. Alternatively- I modified my Savasana for the first 4 years of my son's life to "Mom needs a 10-minute break". When he napped, and as soon as he went to school, and I was able to, what was the first thing I did? Savasana! I truly love and benefit greatly on a regular basis from this pose, heart, heart, heart, heart!!!

And if you find there is still noise in the background, can you just witness it and let it pass?

I am Dead Serious:
<u>If you learn no other yoga pose learn and practice this one</u>!

This pose is truly one of the most challenging. Why? Just look at the way our culture glorifies being busy. I am curious if that is changing...we can hope!

*To come out of the pose, roll onto your side into the fetal position, rest for a few breaths then come up to sitting.

Step by Step - How to Practice Savasana:
-Lay down on the floor, on a yoga mat with a blanket over you
-Set your timer within arm's reach
-Close your eyes

-Lay completely still.

Optional Additions-

Cover your eyes with eye pillow, scarf or cloth, (you can also just close your eyes)

Place a pillow or bolster under your knees, if your lower back feels tight.

You can do this on the floor, in your bed, or on a couch. Ideally here you are able to allow your hands to be loose at your sides.

When the thoughts start crowding in as they will continue to do, practice bringing your mind down into your body. Notice your interior landscape. Scan through your body. Any stiff areas that seem to be holding onto tension, simply ask it to let go? These little spots are waiting for our invitation! Gradually continue to bring your mind back all the way through your body – Surrender to Gravity. You may shift around a little or stretch a little, for example if you roll your head back and forth, see how small of a movement you can make. If you have an itch, it's okay if you scratch, but can you notice it without scratching? Ideally you are to get into a position lying prone and practice to remain completely still for the whole time.

For example:

- Notice the areas of your body touching the surface you are on. Surrender
- from the top of your head, feel your scalp relax, begin to allow the brow to unknit itself and slide back, the eyes soften in their sockets, the jaw slides back, the tongue rests and softens in the mouth.
- You notice the breath. Air moving in and out of your body, without trying to control it. You notice the rise and fall of your chest.
- Your neck and shoulders, let go of all tension,
- You feel your elbows resting on the ground beneath you and your hands roll open.

- Your internal organs are resting inside you, your heart, lungs, stomach, kidneys, intestine, brain, your heavy brain, and all the rest. They are taking care of you all the time. Give them permission to be in a relaxed state.
- When you hear your, hopefully gentle, alarm ring you can stay resting a bit longer then wiggle your fingers and toes before rolling over onto your side and pausing for at least a couple of breaths in the fetal position
- Then bring yourself up to seated

Namaste

At the end of yoga classes, it is customary to place your hands in a prayer-like position, bow slightly and say, "Namaste" (Nah Mah Stay) as a closing farewell acknowledgement. It is a greeting towards yourself, your practice, your instructor and others in the class. It essentially means- The light that dwells in me, bows and acknowledges the light within you. In your own private practice, you can choose to acknowledge this time in practice as well.

Busy Brain Reflection:

This can happen before, during or after Savasana.
Note to self- Do not start rearranging the furniture! What is your go to busy work activity that keeps you away from what you really care about?

For me it is so many things- Furniture rearranging is one of them, but the regular internet surfing and too much shopping, whether I buy anything or not! Those are close runner ups. Another one I'm pretty sure I'm not alone in is – picking on myself. literally physically mentally & emotionally. Physically- my face – Looking at myself under a microscope so to speak, in an anxious moment is a learned behavior I have had to break out of, and it's an ongoing process. The first step of the process is noticing it happening. Well rested mindfulness is the best solution I have found.

Many years ago, I noticed the seriously wrong nature of this but I did not know what to do about it. After many years of inner work with and without professional help I am able to recognize ways to get through it and move forward with life. Hurray! It's taken some practice, but here's what I do- I say "Stop" outloud and coordinate it with the action of taking a step back (from the mirror or whatever the current unwanted activity behavior it is) and say you are alright. And take a deep breath.

Often I have noticed there is voice over going on in my head that isn't always in the right. I have noticed for instance when people say, "oh I like your curly hair", they usually don't actually want curly hair, deep down somewhere in them, they like what they have and that is a good thing. What I mean by this is liking what you have and working with it is liberating. Go with what you've got. You are allowed to like your life! The critical voice will get quieter if you tell it thank you and that it can take a break !

Simplify life to live.

First thing- notice when it's happening- and address it- oh there you go again – take away the inner critic's power by calling it out.
Secondly- Tell them/ yourself to "Stop" the behavior.
If it doesn't work, forgive yourself, and try again next time or start over.
Are you tired? Probably. Overwhelmed with thoughts? This is normal. The thoughts will keep coming, notice if you can let them pass by. If it's important, trust yourself that you will deal with it.

Savasana is a yoga pose about quelling the fears within us about our own finite mortality. Still the Body, Still the Mind. For me it is a way of melting away pain strain, mental physical and spiritual exhaustion, and saying goodbye to overwhelm and starting fresh. In this practice you will literally feel these unwanted things dissolving.

It might be immediate, or it might take some time, but at a certain point in savasana it's like a wave that passes over you and the tiredness and overwhelm goes away, and there, you are ready to take on the rest of your day.

Savasana is rejuvenating, and the closest thing I've found to the fountain of youth. Truly, a real honest to goodness life saver.

*Namaste

3. BREATHING EQUALS LIFEFORCE

The most important element of Yoga.

The Ujjayi (oo-ja- yee) Breath is a breathing technique that translates from sanskrit to the Victorious Breath

Breathing is the most important part of practicing yoga. The way that the Ujjayi breath is practiced is by creating a throttle at the back of the throat.

Breathing- Take a Deep Breath-There's no getting away from it. You can't hold onto it; you have to go through it. Then-let it go- the simplest and yet at times the most challenging practice in life.

There was a difficult time I went through in my life in my early twenties. I would look in the mirror and I looked translucent... I suddenly noticed I wasn't breathing! This was the moment I made the step forward to learning Yoga.
How long can we live without breathing? 2 minutes? Maybe a little longer. The breath is so integral to our lives and we don't even have to think about it.

What happens when we actually focus on the breath?
For me I notice its edges, I notice the lack of breath in my voice at times. I notice my emotions, both joy and distress. Laughter really helps us relax and let the breath pass through. Who else out there loves a good bout of laughter?

Sometimes we hold our breath too, like when we are scared, or worried or nervous.

The most important element of Yoga.

During Yoga practice we can begin to coordinate the movements with the breath and realize how much the in breath and out breath are what sustains us. We need both.

The biggest thing is to begin to notice the breath moving in and out of us, but here is the breathing technique I use during yoga practice. I've practiced and taught it so much that when I go into a yoga session, I automatically go into this type of breathing. It stimulates the vagus nerve, for powerful natural healing and balancing. It focuses us on the present moment and it helps us to develop breath control. The ability to deepen and lengthen our breathing, is life affirming.

The Ujjayi Breath- The Victorious Breath- Inspiration

How to do the Ujjayi Breath.

Turn the corners of your mouth slightly up and in. Gaze softly in front of the tip of your nose.

As you breathe in and out through the nose, create a throttle in your throat. You will know you are on the right track when you hear a wind-like sound swirling around at the back of the throat. It can also be likened a little to the sound of ocean waves how they sound a little bit different rolling in than they do rolling out.

Sometimes it sounds like Darth Vader! Pay attention to the rise and fall of the breath.

We come in to this world, and we will someday leave We are a steady balance of embodied inspiration breathing in life, pausing soaking it in, and letting it go, recognizing with each breath out that yes one day our time will expire- exhalation- and pausing and allowing it to be as it is and will be.

Pranayama is the Sanskrit word for breath work and awareness. Inhale- Exhale and the pauses between. Breath work awareness. Bring your awareness into your body, notice it without judgment and allow it to be, to flow in and out of you.
This in Yoga is known as Prana.

Prana is another word for the Life energy within us.
The very most important aspect of yoga practice.

4. MOUNTAIN POSE

"Tada! Yes, Just Stand There."

Mountain Pose - Tadasana

As I write this, I notice I've been sitting a lot. In a chair. I make a habit of getting up regularly and I am in the habit of starting my writing sessions with the end in mind- Savasana.

As I get up, I walk mindfully to the kitchen to get a drink of water or make a cup of tea. I stand in the kitchen at the counter and bring my attention down through my body to my feet. I notice my posture, I notice how I am distributing the weight and I check to even it out. I notice what is going on for a few quiet breaths. Then I go back to work.

You can also practice this pose sitting in a chair. Using a chair follows the same steps as explained but is in a seated position with the spine upright, and feet flat on the floor.

This is Mountain Pose or Tadasana - it literally is just standing there! It makes me smile as I write this when I think of the prevalence of the opposite in our society- 'Don't just stand there- do something!' Here you don't have to. You stand and are present in the moment. You can find your patience; you can breathe and you can observe. You are ready for whatever comes. Like a mountain, you hold yourself steady.

I practice this pose whenever I have to stand and wait. It's great in lines. As you scan through your body, notice your posture from the ground up. Your legs are passively active, you don't hang back into your knees. You stack your joints from the ankles all the way up to your neck bones.You notice where you might be out of alignment and you adjust to be comfortably upright.

How to practice Mountain Pose- Tadasana
Soften your gaze in front of the tip of your nose.

- o   Distribute the weight evenly across each foot. Are they hip distance apart? How can you tell?
- o   Spread your thumb and pinky finger apart (think hang loose Hawaii) that is the distance you need between your feet. Or one of your feet lengths distance between. Are your feet parallel, or is one foot turned out. Keeping the feet parallel gives stability, and helps with our posture all the way up our body.
- o   Spread out your toes, if you can. Notice if your shoes are constrictive or comfortable? Notice if you are gripping with your toes. Are you leaning forward, locking your knees, collapsing your ankles? Your legs want you to activate them. Looking at how your shoes wearout can give hints on how you habitually tend to stand in Mountain Pose.
- o   As you distribute the weight down into the feet, feel your connection with the ground beneath you. At the same time feel an upward moving energy lifting you upwards and holding you in this standing position.
- o   Are you leaning forward or backwards? Bring yourself back to your center. Imagine there is a string attached to your head gently drawing you upwards.
- o   Place your knees with a very slight bend directly above your ankles, - This keeps the legs gently activated. Avoid sitting back into the knees.
- o   The hips then sit directly above the knees. Tune in here and notice if you are tucking the tailbone in or out, can you find the middle ground? Is your Stomach hanging forward? Are you holding tension in your abdomen? Simply observe What is going on without judgment.

- o   Gently draw the navel in.
- o   Keep your heart as light as a feather. Locate your Rib Cage above your hips. I like to imagine an invisible string attached to the top of my sternum drawing me upwards without sticking my ribcage out, to help keep standing tall.
- o   Observe your Shoulders. Relax them away from your ears, and allow them to slide back and down as you softly lift through your center.
- o   Balance your head on top of your body- It holds some weight, 10-12 pounds! I always find this fact surprising. Practicing Mountain pose helps lighten this load. Bring your ears above your shoulders, with your chin parallel to the ground.
- o   As you stand in Mountain pose continue to observe how your body pulls you in habits of standing in different ways. You will notice how your clothing or accessories affect how you stand. You will notice different feelings come up. These can be physical or emotional. Place yourself in the position of the witness and just stand there! Observe what is going on for you.

I find we often pass by this pose fairly quickly, but every breath you can consciously spend in Tadasana is valuable. This is one of those few moments where we notice our gravitational connection to the earth.

The Gazing Point-
Incidentally the gazing point mentioned at the beginning here has a Sanskrit name. It is called Drishti, and it simply helps us to focus our attention inwards on the breath.

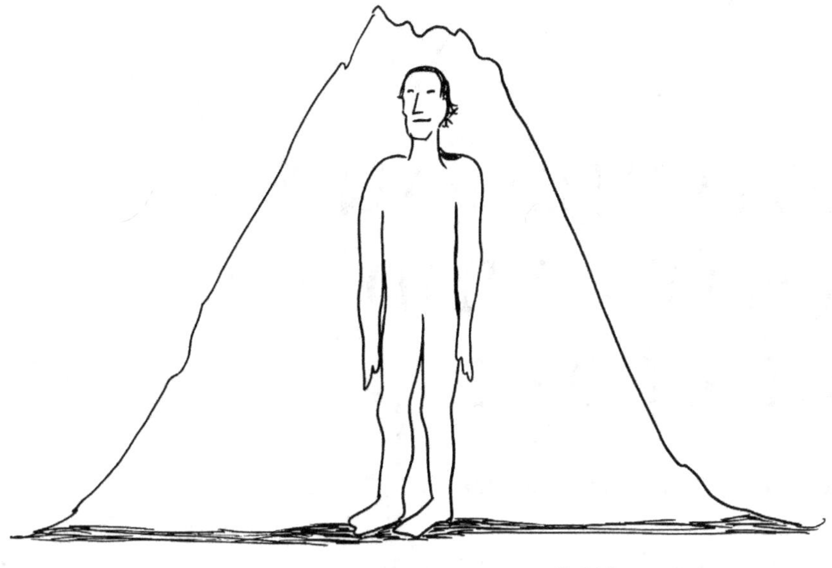

Mountain Pose
Tadasana

5. STRETCH AND CENTER- FIND YOUR CORE

What does it mean to center yourself?

In every practice we begin by centering ourselves. Bringing our awareness to our core, physically and energetically. This of course refers to our core musculature and strength. Also to our central nervous system and the spinal cord, and the energy running up and down it.

Bandhas- Energy Locks

We bring our awareness to our center of gravity at the base of the pelvic floor, over and over again as we practice. This brings a lightness and balance to our practice. It also has a name: Mula Bandha- which means root lock. So we are bringing the energy in as we breathe and holding it steady in our bodies. The next Bandha, called Uddiyana Bandha, is just above the root lock below the navel. When you bring a gentle drawing upward and inward below the belly button, as you practice each pose it can help deepen the experience of your practice. The last one I have learned to focus on is always being aware of keeping your heart lifting and your chin slightly tucked and this is called Jalandhara bandha- All three of these holds, help you to contain the energy of your practice steady in your body with each breath, and gives you something to maintain focus on, always bringing you back to your centerline.

So as the practice goes, once you start breathing, and bring your awareness to your center of gravity, and your navel. Here is a really basic rundown of the Basic yoga pose forms, there are many many variations of each but they boil down to these: Standing poses, Seated poses, & Inversions (equivalent to headstands).

In each practice we will:
Stand Up
Stretch
Sit Down
Put your Feet up
Be with the Child
Lean Back
Look both ways
Lean Forward
Put your Feet up again
Rest

Or in other words: Stand there, sit there, lean in, look both ways, bend over backwards, lean in, turn it around upside down, and let it all go!

Along with breathing through each, that's about it. If you can get this there is no need to read any farther!

For further details and how to settle in and enjoy the process I invite you to please read on.

Something that always kept me interested in yoga was the mind body connection. Yoga is a safe place to experience a sensual part of our nature, we are invited to notice our bodies.
This is not how it was for me to begin with. I thought I knew my body, but I was so disconnected - and so exhausted by trying

to think things through that it took me a while to come into the actual body sense aspects.

Another thing I have noticed is some of the poses we practice in yoga, require a sense of safety- I often remark in my classes that you may be in a vulnerable position but in yoga class you are safe. In yoga class essentially the teacher holds space for the students to experience each pose to the fullest of their ability.

If you find you don't feel safe to lie still for 12 minutes, without being disturbed, perhaps looking into taking a class may be in order.

To stretch is to strengthen, and remember it's not about how deep you can go into a stretch. I cannot emphasize this enough. And that is why I am deciding to make an emphasis on the fantastic modifications we have on the basic yoga poses.

Deciding how to sequence the order of the book. I am giving the reader things they can gradually incorporate into their lives whether they are on or off the yoga mat.

At some point you might just have to stop and get a yoga mat out and practice. It might help to remind yourself, everyone feels better after yoga practice!

The way I was introduced to yoga was gradual and slow. Then I learned a system to instruct that was flowing and vigorous. Because of this I have tended to lead people through a yoga practice as gently as possible. I would also like this to be of practical use to people that they can refer back to this to remember it can be simple. Yoga is about connecting to, noticing, and being where you're at, not about impressing yourself or anyone else with performing some kind of contortionist pose. The more you breathe the deeper you can stretch over time. It's interesting to observe the ebb and flow of how our bodies work.

Avoid comparing yourself to anyone else, avoid fixating images or ideas you may have of what you are supposed to do or look like. Yoga is a safe place to be exactly who you are where you are at, right now at this moment.

For this Book, I am selecting a few simple poses. This way, you or almost anyone can begin a very basic practice without getting overwhelmed. It will be hard for me to limit it, because there are so many great poses you can practice, and one can lead into the next. But the goal here is simplicity. My intuition tells me these are the basics that everyone needs. One can always build on from there, and naturally we are always going back to the basics.

Along with the poses I share in this book will give a lot of focus to modifications. These are ways of doing the pose, where you get all the benefits, without over straining or hurting yourself. <u>It's okay to feel some discomfort but it should not hurt.</u> IF you begin to feel pain, even a little, slowly back out of the pose, come back to a seated position, or Child's pose, which we will discuss in a moment. This is how I originally learned.

Along beside the breathing technique, there is what you call Asana. (sounds like it's written) This is the sanskrit name for the yoga postures or poses. Asana itself is one of the 8 limbs or parts of the study of yoga. Asana is the physical movements of yoga also known as Postures. They were actually originally designed to help prepare one to be able to sit in meditation.

I find asana amazingly provides endless fascination in the subtleties of where we are at any given moment and places to bring our attention and mindfulness to.

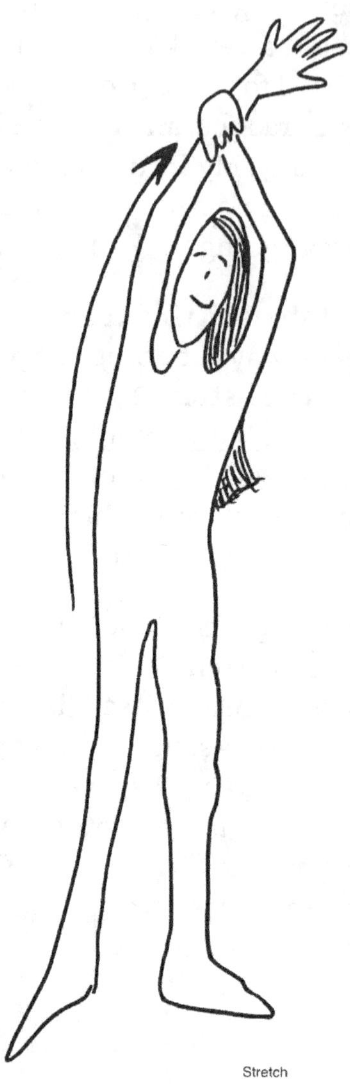

Stretch

6. LEGS UP THE WALL- ONE OF THE BEST THINGS YOU CAN DO

This pose is the definition of Sweet Simplicity,

Coming Down To Earth

I am always amazed at how seldom we in the adult world actually come down onto the actual ground. The ground is good. The ground is stable. The ground supports and connects us.. When was the last time you came down and touched the earth?

Prepare yourself to stay in this pose for 10-20 minutes. You may wish to use a timer.

Amazingly, <u>this pose is one of the single best things you can possibly do</u> for yourself, your body and your overall health.

Practicing Legs up the Wall, reverses the blood flow in the body in a gentle and natural way. It Is a relaxing and calming yet energizing and rejuvenating tonic. It is cleansing too, and because it's a tonic, it has a way of giving us exactly what we need in the moment.

Legs up the Wall or Viparita Karani, basically means Water Fall. Is exactly what it says. Lying on your back with your legs up the wall.

A Simple Inversion, Legs up the Wall is a gentle safe way to get all the same benefits of the more advanced Head stands and Shoulder Stands.

How to do Legs up the Wall
Depending on what is going on with your body you may find it very easy to get into, or you may need a little bit of extra padding like a pillow or folded blanket underneath your hips.

An easy variation is to lie on the floor with your legs up on a chair seat or couch.

At the Wall is best to get the full effect. Essentially Legs up the wall is the easy peasies inversion that is comparable in greatness to headstands and shoulder stands in its health benefits of reversing the blood flow and doing so in the utmost gentle of ways.

Viparita Karani: Getting Situated

Have a pillow, cushion or bolster handy. If you know you have stiffness in your low back or legs or simply for extra comfort, also lay a folded up firm blanket onto the floor at the wall for under your hips. Or just be like a happy little kid and go for it!

With your yoga mat laid out perpendicular, from the wall, sit down at the edge with one shoulder touching the wall.

Using your outside arm for support, lean out from the wall, still keeping your bottom close to the wall, come down to lying on your side.

Roll onto your back and bring your legs up the wall.

Make sure your upper body including your head, is coming straight out from the wall,

Here is where you can also press your legs into the wall, lift your hips and bring the pillow or bolster underneath.

Ahhhhhh! Enjoy!

Stay here, rest and breathe. See if you can focus on your breathing or just watch your mind wander for 20 minutes, you can't go wrong!

The blood, and lymph will flow down your legs and pool in your stomach area and gently continue down your body like a gentle waterfall.

Coming out of the pose:

Take a few minutes to come out of the pose.

- You can take your legs apart in a wide leg spread, straddle position for a few breaths.
- You can take your feet together, knees apart, and bring them down the wall like butterfly wings, for a few breaths.
- Then take your knees together and hug them into your chest.
- Bring your legs back up and then all the way to the side and push yourself up into a seated position.

Notice how you feel.

I have practiced this pose regularly over the years, when I feel exhausted.

Even just the legs on the couch if no wall space is presenting itself is good.

The Main Idea

The main idea is to bring the head below the level of the heart.

I have often wondered why they don't make easy chairs to actually go back far enough to bring the legs above the heart (or farther)? I think it would help so many people if it did!

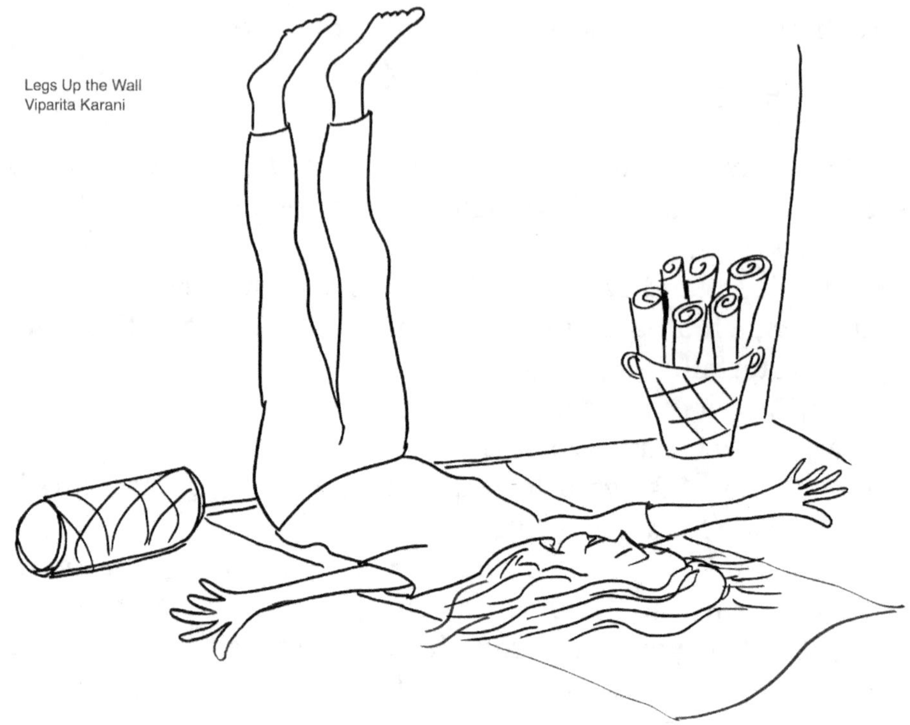
Legs Up the Wall
Viparita Karani

7. CHILD'S POSE

Bow Down And Honor The Child Within, Put Another Way - Rest And Play.

This is not what I would have said when I was first learning yoga. But did we ever do a lot of Child's Pose! Having an attitude of playfulness helps us get the most we can out of this pose.

"Pose of the Child!", my teacher would say, and we would all go down onto our mats with our foreheads down. When I would pop back up, she would say, "Stay in Childs pose and breathe!' As I learned to keep my forehead down, I noticed little things like a small triangle of light back between where my toes met. I noticed a coolness in my body. My forehead felt massaged by the mat. It was so comfortable! And so Child's pose it was!

Child's pose is like a tonic. Child's pose relaxes the muscles on either side of our spine, it helps us with our digestion and it is calming and restful while at the same time being energizing. You will actually see small children automatically go into this pose. Child's pose feels good. Child's pose is fun. And Child's pose prepares us to be able to do other poses.

Sometimes people's legs and hips are tight as they go to rest their hips back. In this case, to get the full experience, you will need to incorporate support. Either under the body- you can lean into and hug forward on a bolster or stack of cushions, or have one wedged between legs and hips as you sit back. It's okay if your hips don't go all the way back to begin with, but make sure you do your best to rest into it.

Another great very simple variation of Child's pose in a chair is this- push your chair back from the table a little way.   Then rest your forehead on the backs of your hands. And breathe!

In all these poses try for 5 to 8 breaths at a time or about 30 seconds- up to 2 or 3 minutes.

Full Child's Pose
1. Come down onto the floor, on your yoga mat or on a carpet with a blanket,
2. Start out on your hands and knees.
3. Check and make sure knees are directly below hips and wrists are directly below shoulders.
4. Sit your Hips back to the heels and bring your big toes to touch.
5. Depending on comfort, you may choose from the following:

- Rest your forehead on to your fists stacked onto of each other or,
- Rest your head onto a firm pillow or bolster or,
- Rest your forehead onto the backs of the hands

Or

- Rest forehead onto the ground in front of you with hands loosely back by your ankles.

To come out of the pose - Place your hands beneath your shoulders and press up to a seated position

Consequently, another pose close to this one is a deeper stretch known as Forward Facing Hero,. This is similar to Child's pose but more active -Here you reach your arms in front of you with your forehead on the floor and your hips back at your heels.

Forward Facing Hero - (Urdhva Mukha Virasana)- Take your calves and knees out to sides and sit hips back between ankles, while you reach and comfortably stretch your arms forward.

Then here follows an even further stretch, depending on the day..

Supta Virasana- From seated lay all the way back - Intense front thigh stretch.

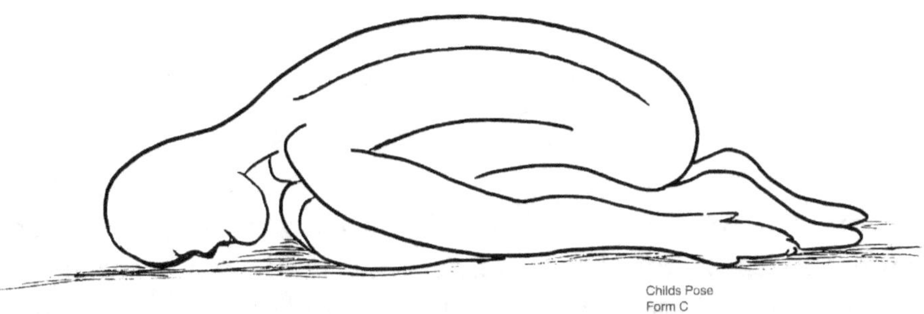

Classic Child's Pose/ Balasana

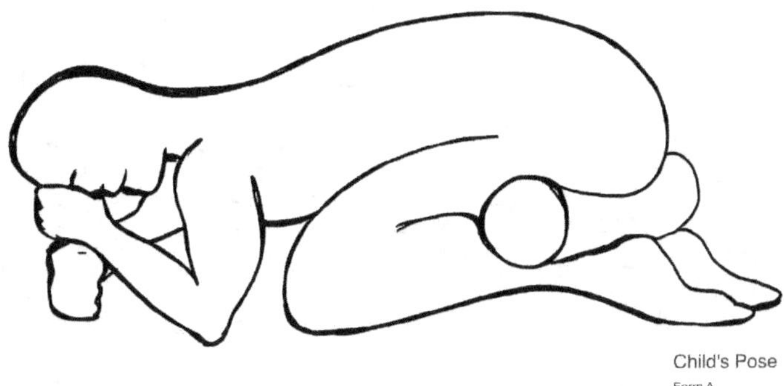

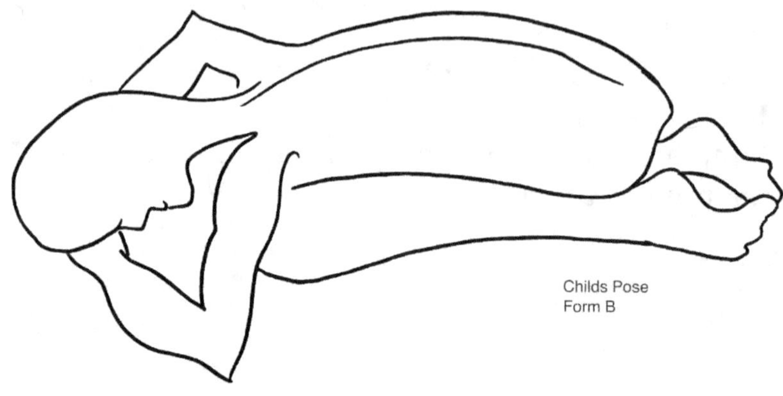

Childs Pose
Form B

Forward Facing Hero is a really good stretch . If you try it, remember to widen your shoulders back and away from your ears while you press your hands into the ground and pull back through your hips.

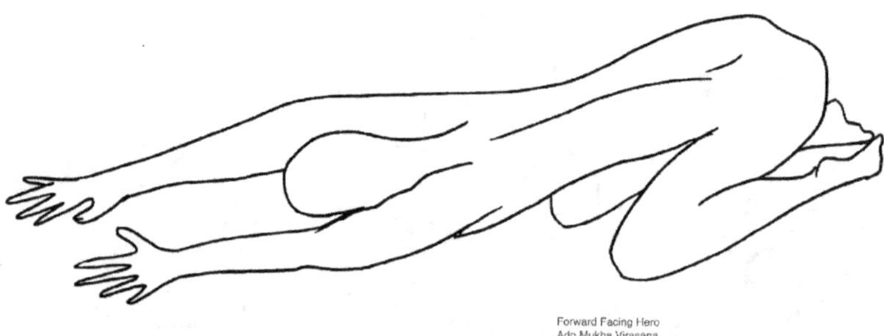

Forward Facing Hero
Ado Mukha Virasana

I find it curious but not surprising that child's pose and hero pose are so similar.

8. STRETCHING LIKE CATS & DOGS

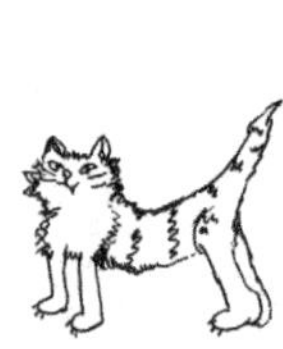 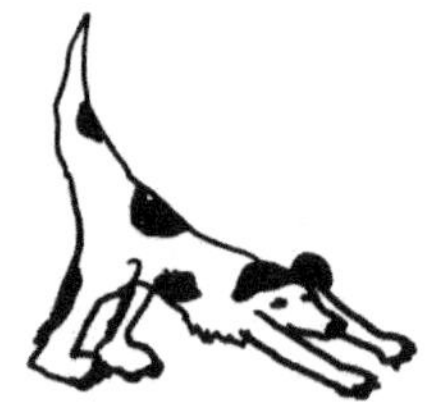

Much better than fighting!

Cat Stretch

Next time you find yourself on the floor- like now? Find a surface that doesn't kill the knees.

Line your knees up under your hips
Line your wrists up beneath your shoulders.
First let your tummy sag down
Next arch your back up like a cat!

Repeat this slowly several times.
Emphasize breathing in when you let your tummy sag and your heart lift. Also look upwards
and lift the tailbone while extending back. Fill your lungs with oxygen.
Emphasize breathing out when you let your back arch upwards. Press into your hands evenly,
with fingers spread wide apart, release your head downwards, and look back between your knees.Tuck your

tailbone under.

Downward Facing Dog Pose- From Cat Stretch
I see dogs stretch like this all the time- I used to have a little dog and when she did it I would say "Adho" For the name of the pose Adho Mukha Svanasana- This actually trained her and she would do the pose on command. She loved it!

Imagine you have a long tail like a dog, and you're ready to play!
From all fours, spread your fingers wide,
straighten your arms and legs at the same time and lift your hips up and back.
It's okay to have a bend in the knees, and breathe into the backs of the legs!
Keep lifting the hips,
Pressing down with the arms,
Alternate between coming high up onto the balls of the feet,
And letting the heels fall back to the floor.
Feet do not have to be flat on the floor.
This is a very active pose, and it stretches the whole back side of the body.

A lot of people have tension and stiffness in the backs of the legs.
If and when it becomes too much of a stretch,
Or even if it doesn't, especially when you are learning,
Alternate back into Child's pose and rest. Yes you have permission to rest .

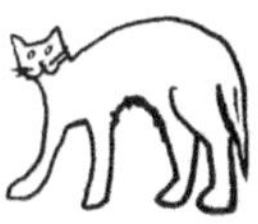

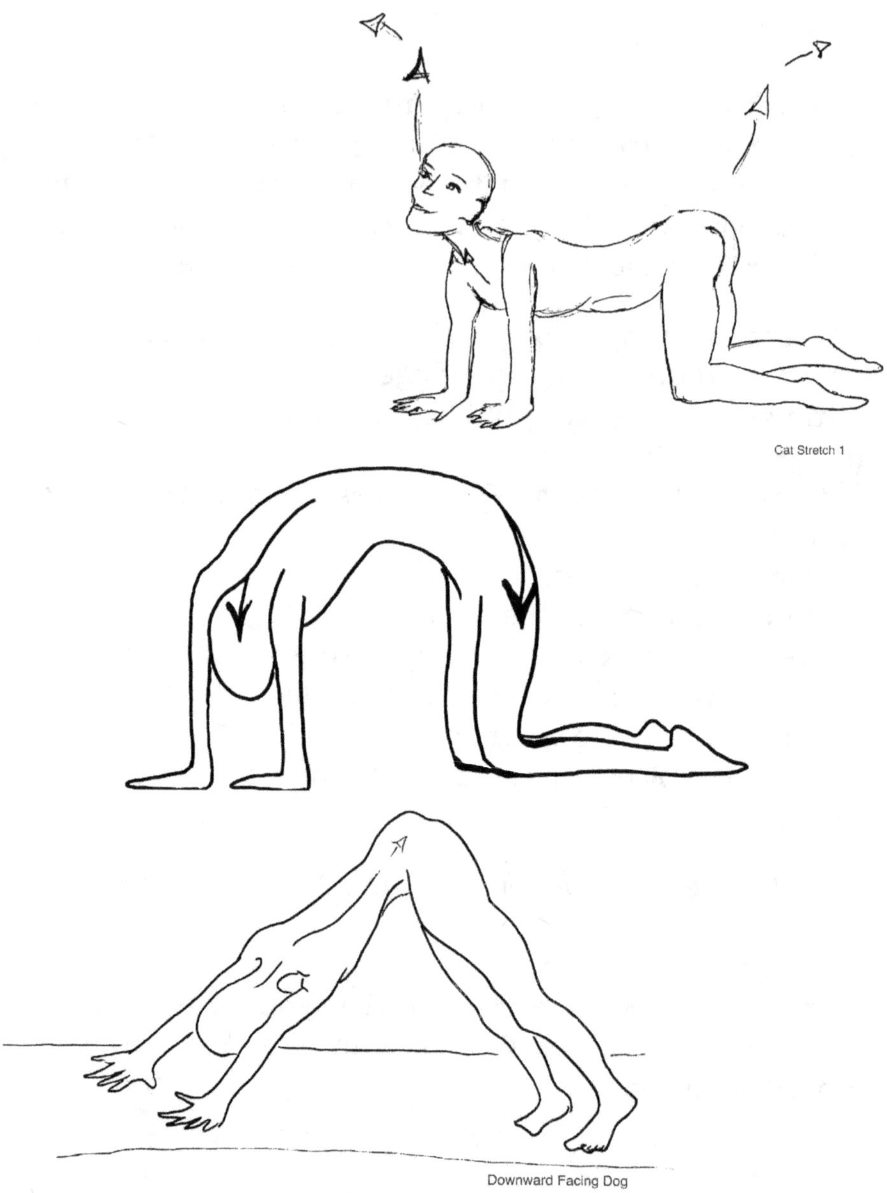

Cat Stretch 1

Downward Facing Dog

9. CROCS & COBRAS

Cooling Down and Rising Up

The Evolution From Crocodile To Cobra.

Crocodile pose gives a feeling of calming safety and groundedness, you feel a great connection to the earth and it is restful. Cobra is energizing to the nervous system, in a grounding way, because although it is a back bend. The legs stay on the ground and you are rooted to the ground by your pubic bone.

Lie down on your tummy with your forehead resting on the backs of your hands. This is the pose of Crocodile

Feel the comfort and calming and breath as you rest here. Feel the whole front of your body completely grounded to the earth.

Cobra Pose
Next when you are ready, come up onto your elbows, line them up directly below your shoulders so your forearms are at approximately a right angle, with your hands extended in front of you and your fingers spread wide.
Press your hands in and lift slightly, pulling forward from the pubic bone down into the ground. Tighten your buttocks a little and draw your spine forward. Allow your shoulders to slide down while your spine lengthens forward and you activate the legs behind you.
Take 5 to 8 breaths,

You can alternate between Crocodile and Cobra a couple of times. This is an energizing back bend so when you are done, it will feel really good to go into Child's pose for a few breaths with your knees bent and your head down on your mat or bolster.

Upward facing dog- WARNING This is a deeper backbend- if Cobra was intense, you can leave this one out. Be sure to keep the buttocks tightened to help protect the low back. On the other hand you might just feel naturally like going into it. Remember to keep your heart as light as a feather, chest lifting and open, and as in all poses- breathing deeply!

Upward facing dog From Cobra pose, press your hands into the ground, straighten your arms and bring yourself forward and up.
Legs stay active, heart is lifting, eyes gaze towards your brow.
Shoulders relax back and down, chest is opening and you are breathing. Deepening into the pose with each inhale.
Stay in the Upward dog until you know you've gotten 1 really good comfortable deep inhale.
Then- you can either go back into Child's pose or roll back over the toes, lift your hips up and back and go into Downward facing Dog.
Spread your shoulders wide and roll your arms to the outside and reach through the arms into the ground..
Let your heels drop back towards the floor here, and feel the stretch in the backs of the legs. If the hamstrings are really tight it's fine to bend the knees and continue to stretch the hips up high.

Take 5-8 breaths here
When ready come back down into child pose for a rest any time.

You can also go into downward dog from Child's pose- hands reach forward, toes turn under, tailbone lifts high and back up in the sky.

Crocodile & Cobra

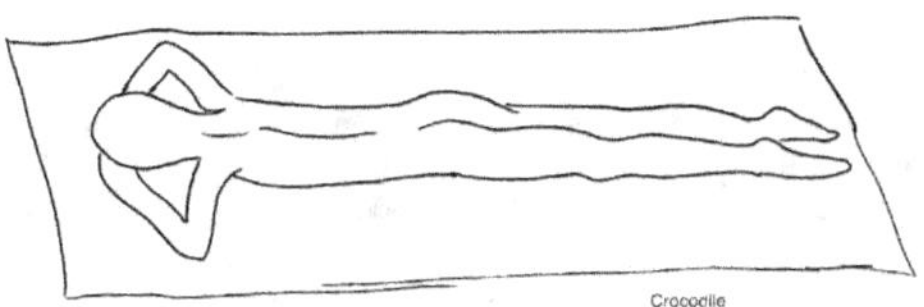

Crocodile

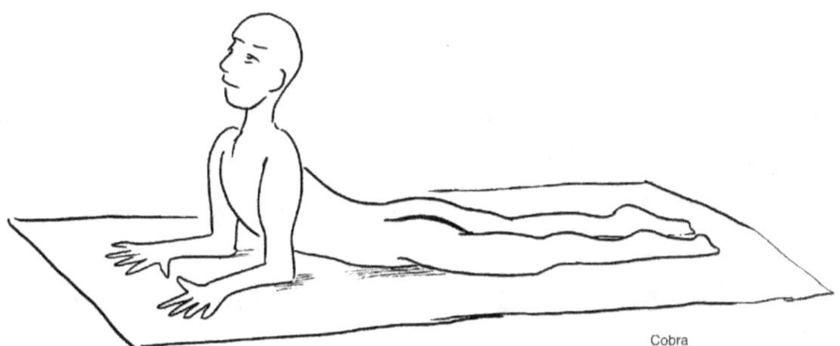

Cobra

10. LOOK BOTH WAYS - WITH A TWIST

Everybody loves a good twist thrown into the story.

Twists are great for squeezing fresh oxygenated blood through your internal organs. They are detoxifying, cleansing and toning like wringing out a wet rag. Seated ones are great between forward bends.

Being gentle and incorporating your whole spine up to the top of your head is key. Even include gazing out the corner of your eyes over your shoulder as part of the movement, and of course breathe as you deepen with each exhale. Inhale lift the spine, exhale rotate.

Chair Twist

I think many people may be familiar with the chair twist. Sit sideways in a chair with a back. Inhale, sit tall, exhale, turn towards the back of the chair and look out over the shoulder.

Remember to keep relaxing your shoulders down away from your ears. It's okay to notice your stiffness and be gradual in your movement, incorporate your eyes into the twist, and gently with soft eyes, observe how far over the opposite shoulder you can see without straining. Feet stay flat on the floor.

Marichyasana- Seated Twist

Sit with your right knee upright, and your other leg extended out in front of you. Inhale, reach up and sweep your right hand to behind you flat on the floor, exhale. Inhale reach your left hand up to the sky, pause and then bring your left elbow to the outside of your upright knee.

Inhale, lift the spine, exhale gently, lift up from your hips on the ground, lift and turn to look over your right shoulder. Inhale, fill the lungs with breath, exhale, twist. Hold and breathe gently moving deeper with each exhale for 5-8 breaths.

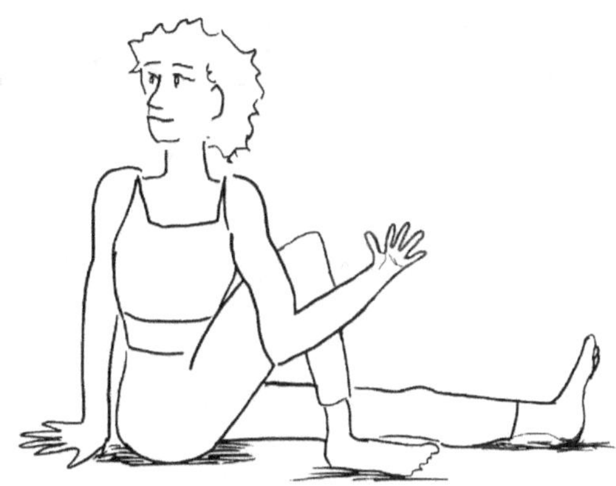

Marychyasana -

Sage Twist

Reclined Twist- Lying Down On The Floor Twist

- Lying on your back hug one knee into your chest.
- Lift your head and bring your chin to your knee, then lie back and draw the knee across the midline of the body.
- While you extend the opposite arm to the side, look out over the shoulder.
- After five to eight breaths, come back to center,
- and then cupping the knee allow it to fall out open to the

same side, and gaze over the opposite shoulder.
- Finally, take the bent knee and either grab the big toe extending the leg upward, lift your chin to your knee, then lay back and allow the leg to fall out to the same side.
- If holding the toes is too much just hold the back of the leg with both hands and when you open out to the side keep the knee bent and cradled in your hand

One last variation that leads us into the next chapter;
Bend one knee and extend the other leg in front of you.
Reach up and forward, and bring you the same side arm back against your upright knee. Press the other hand into the floor and draw yourself deeper into the bent leg Forward bend. Do both sides.

11. FORWARD BENDS

The luxurious supertonic of the forward bend.
Try one today!

Seated Forward Bend- Paschimottanasana

(Pah-shee-moh-tah-nah-sah-nah)

Forward Bending is calming and soothing to our whole systems. We fold forward and let it all go. We ease forward at the hips and squeeze in at the groin area.

Because of tightness in the backs of the legs, many people need to warm up to this one.

Holding a strap looped around the feet can help stretch out those pesky hamstrings.

Even easier and just as effective, is to simply bend the knees as you fold forward!

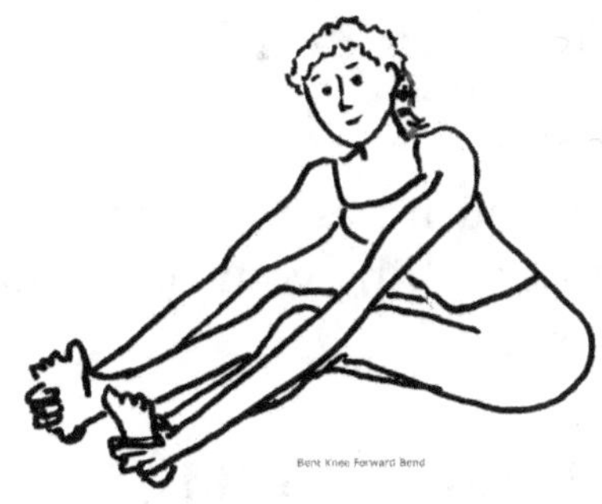

Bent Knee Forward Bend

Focus on extending the spine up and forward while you rest into it, to get the most benefits. It doesn't matter if you can reach your toes!!

Dandasana is the name of the starting point pose - it is in fact a simple forward bend.

Starting out with the feet and legs actively extended straight out in front of you, and your hands at your sides on the floor.

Paschimottanasana- Seated Forward Bend. Take a deep inhale and reach up to the sky- look up and extend your spine upwards. Now as you exhale, lengthen your spine forward and bend at the hips. Reach casually for your feet- the key here is to not worry too much about reaching the feet but more about lengthening the spine.

-You can bend the knees
-You can use a strap around the feet,
-You can truly be content with your hands on your knees

Focus on the breath moving you gradually deeper with each exhale, into the bend at the hips.

This pose flushes your deep lower abdominal organs with fresh oxygenated blood and is very calming.

Enjoy this pose for 5 to 8 breaths. Remember a breath is an inhale as well as an exhale!

Deep Forward Bend

Extension -
If you find it easy to go into a deep forward bend, as some people do, touching your toes is no problem? Then you can add 3 variations.

1 - Hold Onto Your Big Toes Look Up Breathe In And Then Draw Yourself Deeper 5-8 Breaths

2 - Hold onto the sides of your feet- lift your heart, look up with a deep inhale, then exhale as you surrender forward. Take 5-8 breaths.

3 - On the third time - From Dandasana, reach for the sky with a deep inhale, then reach forward and grasp a hold of your wrist as you fold deeply into the forward bend. You can rest your forehead onto your knees.

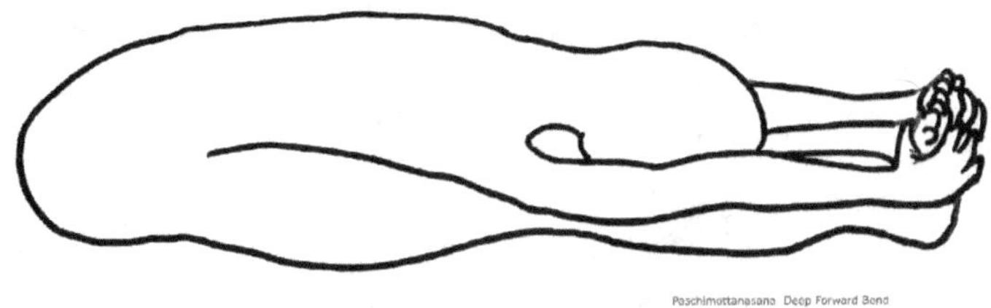

Paschimottanasana Deep Forward Bend

Bathtub Bending

I find one of the most soothing and simple things to connect, cleanse and soothe yourself to the center of our bones and being is a bath.

Bending becomes easier too! Next time you are able to get into the tub or other body of water, notice how well you are able to ease more deeply into a forward bend.

As gratitude would have it, I had the good fortune of living in a place one time which had a large old fashioned clawfoot tub. This is where I really began to establish the enjoyable ritual of bathing for relaxation that I return to again and again. The tub would warm up and stay warm for a long time and you could fill it really deep. It was exquisite.

Since then, in all the places I have lived, I have never again encountered another tub quite like that one yet. But I have found that even in the smaller versions of bathtubs out there, right down to soaking the feet in a washtub, one can enjoy the simple soothing magic of immersing yourself in water.

Epsom salts are a very soothing addition for sore muscles. While you're at it, why not throw in a few handfuls of baking soda? It's a beautiful recipe for relaxation.

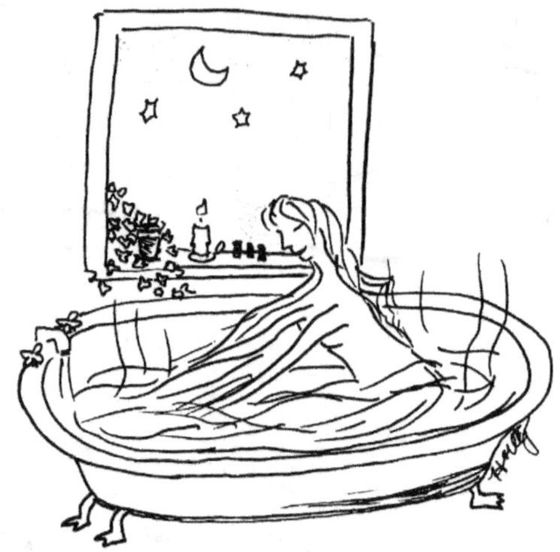

Standing Forward Bends- Padangusthasana-
Standing, bend forward. bend forward for 5 to 8 breaths and notice how you can deepen into it.
Does it feel tight?- Bend the knees. This enables you to lengthen the spine.

Here are 3 standing modifications to help your body get into a good forward bend are this- use a table top or the wall to support you.

1. Lay with your upper body on a table with your legs from the hip crease hanging down to the floor, standing or taking the weight off the feet. It feels really good !
2. With your hands on a Table top- leave them there flat and now step back a leg's distance from the table, bend at the hips, press into the ground with your feet and extend

back through the tailbone.

3. The Wall- the same as above but you start with your hands and body close to the wall and then walk out until you are bent at a right angle- more or less. Remember to bend the knees, and keep pushing in through the feet as you extend back through your tailbone- At the same time press into the wall with your hands a shoulder's distance apart and your shoulders relaxed and spread aways from your ears.

It's like you are making your back into a table top.

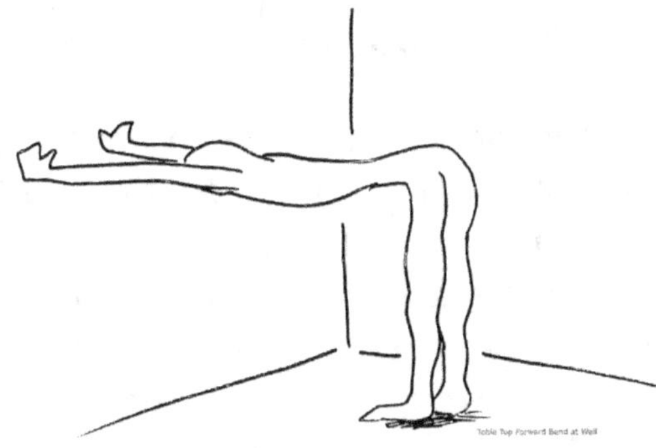

12. VINYASA - THE CONNECTIVE SEQUENCE.

Putting It All Together With Vinyasa

Vinyasa simply means connective sequence. Ashtanga Yoga, also popularly known as Power Yoga is what I was first trained to instruct. It is a specific sequence of poses in a specific connected order that synchronizes with the breath. There are a number of series of them that go from quite accessible to more and more pretzel-like difficulty. I have been trained mainly in the first and some in the second series, but "The Primary Series" is all that has really been necessary in my life path or in teaching, so far.

Occasionally a pose from the second series will be incorporated into the primary series. What I have always found very fascinating about Ashtanga Yoga is how well concentration on the continuous Ujjayi breath heated up the body and led you to greater flexibility. I also always found it novel how well all the poses of the series moved into the next. Ashtanga yoga is a vigorous style of yoga.

From my own experience, I am grateful that I had taken other yoga classes *before* learning the alignment of the poses separately and gradually. However I am influenced by my power yoga training background, and you may notice this book is arranged in such a way that you can go from pose to pose in a vinyasa type sequence. One Important challenge to remember is to slow down. *Yoga is not aerobics*. Breathe and remember often - less is more!

This little sequence of moves along with the breath, will heat you up and allow your muscles to bend and move. As I was taught, just like iron when heated will bend, so will the body with the breath.

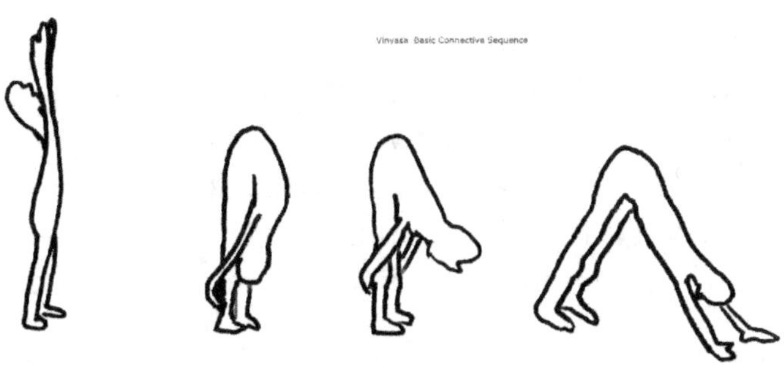

Sun Salutation - Surya Namaskara

Stand There, in mountain pose.
Reach for the sky -Inhale!
Look up
Bend forward – Exhale
Look at your navel-
Lift your head, and look up to your brow- Inhale

Step back into a plank (push-up) position
  Lower down to towards the ground
  Roll Forward on your toes, straighten your arms,
  Lift your heart and your gaze into Upward facing dog - Big Inhale then as you exhale,
  Roll back over your Toes
  Lift your hips up high towards the sky-
  Hold here for 5 full breaths.
  (or take a rest in child's pose)
  Next, step or hop looking forward-with a big Inhale,
  then surrender your head down with and exhale,
  Finally with an inhale come back up to standing
  Reach hands up together above your head
  And exhale and bring your arms back down to your sides.

Or from hips in the air, come through to seated, with legs extended in front.
  Or come down onto hands and knees and into Child's pose to rest.

Repeat 5 times (this takes about 15 minutes)

Now be sure to make time to have a "12-minute Break" Savasana to soak it all in.
  You can also use it as a warm up to then move into the other poses in the booklet.
  If you coordinate the movements with the breath I can assure you, you will warm up.
  You will bend.

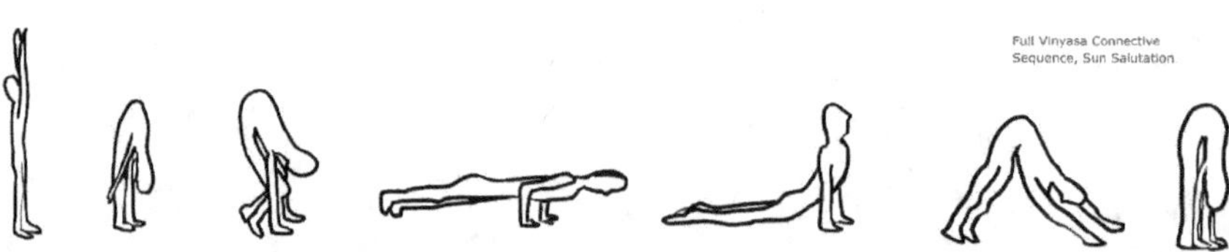

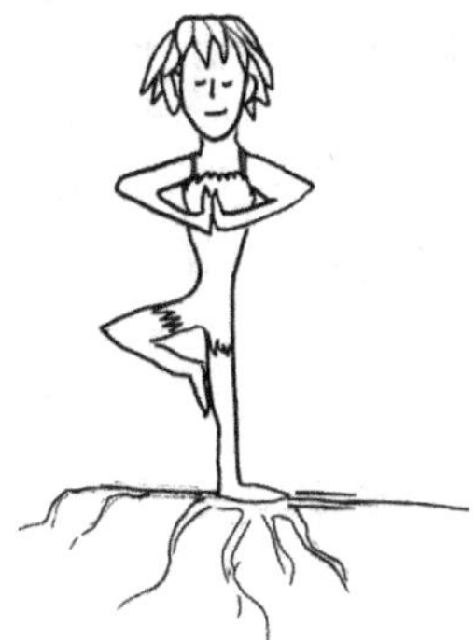

Tree Pose- Vrksasana

13. BE THE TREE

Tree Pose- Vrksasana

Meet me back at the kitchen counter here. (Or of course your yoga mat at the wall!) Maybe the kettle is boiling.

From Mountain pose, choose a spot in front of you that isn't going to move to hold your gaze. This will help you hold your balance.

Bring one foot slowly up to your leg just above the knee. Press your foot into the leg, and equally press your leg back into your foot.

You can use the kitchen counter or wall to hold onto or see if you can balance for 5 inhales and exhales.

Now do the other side. Is one side easier than the other?

As we move into more poses that stretch one side of the body. Prepare yourself to always be in the habit of doing both sides.

Tree pose is fun because it is a good feeling when we can find our balance, and it brings us back to our childhood when we can't!

14. CLEANSING FROM THE INSIDE OUT.

Depending on what we do, eat, or environments we find ourselves in our eating and lifestyle habits, or even the work environment can create build ups in our systems. For a few examples maybe you have to work where there is too much dust, or it's the season of extra pollen counts in the air. Maybe you've been in a cycle of eating extra amounts of processed foods or refined flours, somethings that become toxic in our systems we may ingest inadvertently or on purpose. Maybe it's too much sugar, dairy or a little too much alcohol, too habitually often. The way I see it, too much of anything isn't good for us. Even broccoli! Have you been eating too much broccoli lately?

Have you been working around the clock? Too much awake timep?

I find all these things can make my system feel stuffy, groggy, lethargic and heavy or bloated. When stuff builds up in our system, what can we really do? Here are a couple of ideas that really do work when you are feeling bogged down.

Cleansing 101- Introducing The Neti Pot

As I have said, the most important aspect of Yoga is - The Breathing

But what do you do if you can't breathe? What if you're all stuffed up? This was actually a huge question I had for many years.

I grew up with terrible allergies and asthma. When I started learning yoga, I was always out of breath, had low energy and could not breath through my nose, which I felt helpless and ashamed about. That was 25 years ago.

At that time, I had gone through a difficult time. I was feeling terrible and could not seem to get out of feeling depressed about how a roommate living situation had worked out. During this time, I noticed one day I was having trouble seeing myself in the mirror- like I was fading away! I realized I wasn't breathing and it occurred to me, since I was in the city that I would look into taking some yoga classes, because somehow, I knew yoga was one thing related to breathing, so that's what I did.

I still remember the teacher getting us to do Child's pose and breathe! And get up and do standing poses and Breathe! I would apologize that I couldn't breathe through my nose and she would say that doesn't matter, just Breathe! So, through the mouth it was for the first while.

Breathing is more important than any pose you do in yoga.

When I found myself in a yoga instructor program a few years later, I learned of a valuable cleansing technique which involves using something called a Neti Pot.

Neti Pot is a technique where you pour lukewarm sea salted water from a little pot with a spout, through your nasal passages.

People tend to shy away a little from this one because it is a bit wet and messy. In western society, for some reason we can tend to get uncomfortable about our bodily functions. But it doesn't have to be this way! I want to share this one with you because knowing a couple of tips that were taught to me helped me get over the discomfort and it is a technique I go back to again and again. It helps with allergies, balances the left and right side of the brain, and can even save you from getting sick!

And I love that you don't even need an actual Neti pot! As shared with me by a really nice yoga teacher in Calgary named David McAmmond. Here's How:NETI POT INSTRUCTIONS

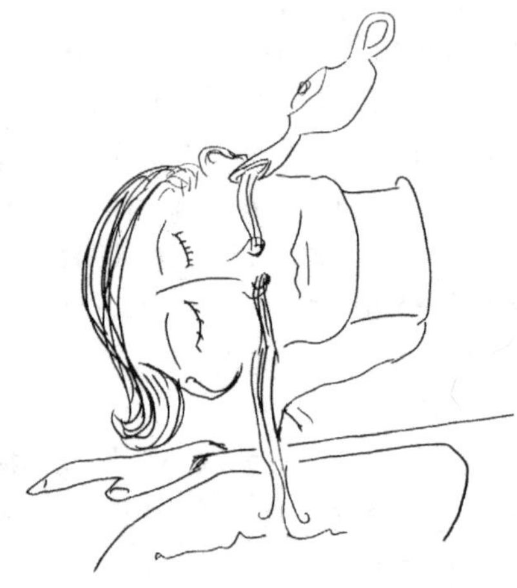

What you need is Sea Salt and <u>Lukewarm, body temperature water</u>, not too hot, not too cold, you feel like the water running out of the tap feels the same as the temperature of your hand. That's the key!

-If the salt water is too cold or hot it can sting a little. Taking the time to make the water feel the exact same temperature of your hand will eliminate the stinging and make you more likely to use the technique.

-If you have a Neti pot, you then add a small spoonful of salt around a ¼ teaspoon.or about 1.5 grams. Stir it to dissolve.

-Then over the sink tilt your head sideways parallel to the sink and place the spout at the upper nostril, relax and ….wait. Here is a place where you may need to exercise a bit of patience and you may be breathing through the mouth.

-Wait until the water starts to flow out of the other nostril. You pour half the pot through and switch sides, or do two pot fulls it's up to you.

-You can blow out your nose into a tissue between the sides.

Neti With A Soup Bowl

Don't have a Neti pot?
-No problem! You may still enjoy the benefits of Neti pot technique -without a Neti pot.
You will still need Sea Salt and Lukewarm, body temperature water and a sink.
You will also need - a soup bowl.

- Take the time to make the water the temperature of your own skin, let it pour it into the bowl, add and dissolve the salt.
- Now take the bowl in front of you and dip your nose into the edge of the bowl of water.
- Over the sink now sniff in steadily, as if you are drinking the water in through your nose, and spit the salt water out of your mouth into the sink.

By relaxing and allowing the warm salt water to flow through will gently clear, moisturize and cleanse your sinus passages.

I find it is great in the cold season. If there is a mucus build up. Or for dealing with allergies you can try it to effectively clear out what is triggering the reaction.

As a side note; I made a point of teaching my baby to get used to gently sniffing a little warm water from his bath through his nose. I would even occasionally add a pinch of sea salt if I thought he might be coming down with something or if I noticed sniffles coming on and I am happy to say at age seven he has hardly ever been sick!

Now I know what to do when I have trouble breathing, I check in with myself. Am I clogged up? Am I forgetting to breathe? Or is it staggered and shallow? Check in and ask, "Am I just tired and exhausted?" Sometimes admitting how tired we might be is difficult, you may just need to wind down, take yourself out of the current situation and put yourself to bed.

Sleep helps restore regular breathing too.

Sweet Dreams

Fire Breathing

Fire breathing cleanses in a more gentle, less watery manner. Sitting comfortably, on a straight backed chair or cross legged on the floor, Press your hands into the floor or chair seat. Lift off slightly if you can and as you draw your tummy inwards with each breath puff the air out of your nose in an outward sniffing manner for 25 breaths. At the end take a long exhale and long inhale or 5 and rest.

This one is usually done at the end of the ashtanga Yoga Series, and right before Savasana.

The Lions Pose!

I will leave you at the conclusion here with a funny one! You could say it's quite simple to do too. It is also powerful! According to Light on Yoga, It cleanses the body of toxins, helps with halitosis/bad breath, even stammering AND it gives us courage. Here's how you do it:

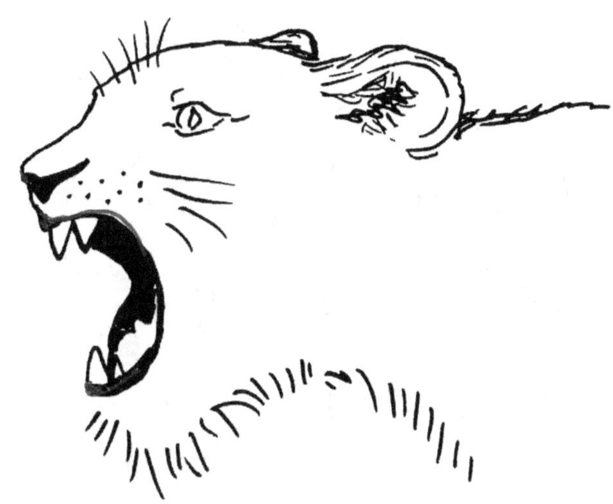

Lions Pose

All at the same time:
Roll your eyes upward,
Stick out your tongue
as far as it will go,
Open your hands wide
on your lap. Or on all fours,
come through your hands
And roar like a lion.
Repeat this 3 times or more.
ROAR! ROAR! ROAR!

15. YOGA NIDRA-WAKING SLEEP

The Definition Of R & R

At the end of your practice you will go back to your mat and practice ideally 10-20 minutes of Savasana.

An alternative to savasana, would be the practice of Yoga Nidra.

What is Yoga Nidra? Well it is the guided aspect of savasana. Otherwise known as guided relaxation. You can find guided yoga nidra online on you tube. And it usually goes something like this:

Let your breath rise and fall naturally.

Starting at the right thumb simply and methodically scan through your body, giving awareness to each and every body part, without going to sleep:

You can find different versions of this same sequence of yoga on Youtube, so you can get comfy and just allow yourself to listen and be guided through. The idea is to stay awake and you will find yourself taken into the state between being asleep and awake. It is most relaxing and rejuvenating and teaches us the valuable lesson of relaxation.

The sequence can vary but you can expect it to be more or less as follows:

First Notice what you hear, and settle in as you scan, with your internal awareness through your body.

Right Thumb, pointer finger, middle finger, ring finger, little finger, back of hand, front of hand, wrist, forearm, elbow, upper arm, back of shoulder, front of shoulder, armpit, inner right side of body, right hip, right upper leg, right lower leg, right foot, right big toe, second toe, third toe, fourth toe and little toe.

Left Thumb, pointer finger, middle finger, ring finger, little finger, back of left hand, front of left hand, back of wrist, front of wrist, outer forearm, inner forearm, outside of upper arm, shoulder, inner upper arm, inside of left side of torso, left hip, back side of upper left leg, front of left leg, back of left lower leg, top of left lower leg, back of ankle, front of left ankle, left foot, left big toe, left second toe, middle left toe, fourth toe on left foot, left

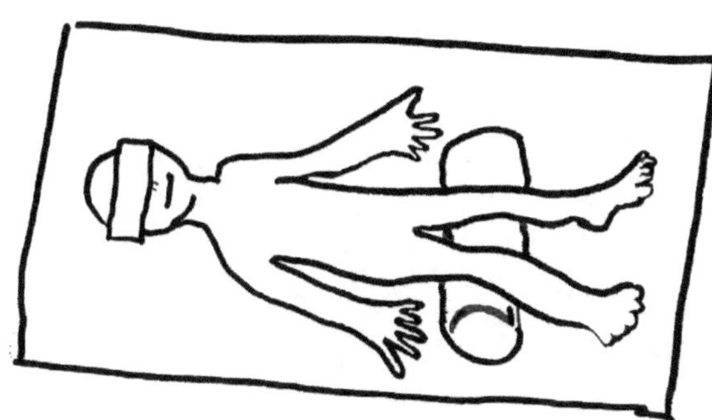

little toe.

Back of head, front of head, forehead and face, right eye, left eye, right nostril , left nostril, right cheek, right ear, left cheek, left ear, lips, chin, throat, back of neck, front of chest, back of chest, lower back, stomach, lower belly, pubic bone and tailbone.

Even reading through it can be relaxing!

Enjoy the stillness of your body, and the subtleties of your body lying still in space, When you are ready to come back into the room, wiggle the fingers and toes, roll to your side and come back up to a seated position.

Now go enjoy the rest of your day.

16. YOGA IS NOT A RELIGION

What is the big idea here?

You are allowed to believe whatever you choose and you can still practice yoga. Since a large part of yoga practice is uniting body, mind and soul. Yoga practice is free from religion, you can bring your own, or not. It has its roots in ancient India, and links to Hinduism The interesting thing is while it really is more of a science, it can bring us to places of knowing our very soul.

I have always loved that yoga is not a religion.

Contemplation now begins. I am going to go a bit into some of my own ideas in relation to our spirit, Ultimately:

Yoga is not a Religion- It is an ancient science, finding interconnection between body, mind and spirit.

But that word Spirit- how can we make sense of this? Well one simple way is to relate the word to Inspiration- or *Inspiritus*- the breath that moves in our body and gives us life.In Yoga

From my own searching and experiences I will share a few thoughts here with you now.

So What is the big idea with Yoga?

Yoga actually means Union or yolk. We become one with the universe or we already are and we become more aware of it, and continue to deepen this awareness through our life practices.

Through its practice you can strengthen and balance not only your physical body but you can begin to experience and feel a force greater than yourself. You begin to recognize the various layers of your being like for example how your mind truly is not exactly who you are

Okay I can get a bit bogged down here in this. I feel as though I am entering a gray foggy unknown area and I'd like to investigate where I'm at here and shed some light to expose the fears and shadows that reside within.

I must admit I feel a wee bit of fear speaking of this. I feel I will be rejected for what I say and persecuted, by all sides! From having interests in Universal Cosmic energy and how it relates to God to having curiosity and interest in studying and learning more about scripture, Christian in particular. There are a lot of strong opinions out there!

My hope is that by shedding light on a few of my own feelings around the subject, fears will lessen their hold and it will lead ever more in the direction of light and love for everyone and everything.

The beauty of Yoga in my opinion, is that because it is about finding inner peace, with yourself, it can unite us all.

In the world there are all kinds of people and circumstances. People can be underhanded, they can lie and cheat you. We live in a place where evil actually exists. Families break up. There are rapists, murderers and there are thieves. Let us remember the fact that there are also generous, kind, caring and sensitive people. While there are all kinds of people, personalities, souls and purposes. We are all different and unique, and the reality is, we are all a little bit the same too.

We could consider that we have a small mind and a big mind

and unfortunately often the small mind seems to win. When I was little, I was told I had an overactive imagination. Now that I'm not so little I realize, this wasn't exactly right. It now seems to me it is actually our own fears of the truth, and the emotions we attach to everything that keep us locked and bound. Becoming aware of this is the first giant step to understanding it and literally changing the world.

Sometimes as I look back at my life, I feel like I have lived a thousand lifetimes. I have thought about these things for a long time and still have trouble putting it into words. Many spiritual concepts are in fact beyond words.

The following is the basic outline of the philosophy behind deepening into yoga practice, paraphrased from B.K.S. Iyengars's book "Light on Yoga". It was believed to be outlined by Patanjali, a realized ancient sage and the proponent of Yoga Philosophy. He was a mysterious wise persona, or could have been more than one person, who wrote the Yoga Sutras - 185 terse aphorisms on yoga. He also wrote a treatise on grammar and on medicine. Here are the eight limbs of practice for inner peace and a brief description.

The Eight Limbs Of Yoga:

1.Yamas - External ethical disciplines - abstinences or universal moral commandments, transcending creeds, countries, age and time
- Ahimsa -nonviolence- non harming other living beings / kindness.
- Satya- Truth (with kindness),
- Asteya- Non-Stealing, including practicing giving credit for ideas too.
- Brahmacharya: continence chastity, this can also mean marital fidelity, and ability to practice sexual restraint (containment)

·   Aparigraha- non-attachment. non-coveting, non-avarice, non-possessiveness- Being able to let go of our attachment to things in the world.

Awareness and practice of the above helps in individual personal growth.

2. Niyamas - Internal Disciplines- Observances-

- Shaucha-purity,
- Santosha-contentment,
- Tapas-persistence, perseverance, self discipline,
- Svadhyaya-Study: of self, reflection, introspection of thought, speech and action
- Ishvarapranidhana - contemplation of God/ Supreme Being,

3. Asana - Posture (meditation seat) - yoga postures, practicing without strain to be able to sit comfortably with chest, neck and head upright in meditation.

4. Pranayama - Breath control - Inhalation, pause, Exhalation, pause.

5. Pratyahara - Withdrawal of senses- consciously choosing to withdraw senses from the outside world and turning to the inner wisdom within.

6. Dharana - Concentration- practicing for instance bringing focus back to your breathing helps train our mind from jumping around.

7. Dhyana - Meditative absorption-nonjudgmental observation. Being in the place of the witness. Watch the thoughts, emotions and feelings rising up, coming and going, and moving through without following them. Yes it takes practice!

8. Samadi - Union, integration- absorption- All coming together into the step beyond meditation, which is beyond words, described as bliss & superconsciousness. You know like when things are ALL GOOD.

Referenced from Iyengar Light on Yoga,

BKS Iyengar c.1991

While yoga is not a religion, the eight limbs suggest further deepening our practice by including the study of scripture.

Religious Scripture And Books

There are lots of books on yoga, spirituality and religion. These include but are certainly not limited to: The Bhagavad Gita story of Arjuna and Krishna of Hinduism, Siddhartha the story of Buddha , books by various Yogis like Paramahansa Yogananda who wrote Autobiography of a Yogi, was sent by his lineage to prove unity between eastern and western religions, and Swami Rama, who not without controversy, wrote Light on superconscious meditation.

As far as scripture goes, I have even come to revisit the scripture of my upbringing- the Bible. Undeniably a compelling complex, cryptic and profound set of works holding plenty of potential for contemplation. This doesn't exclude other forms of scripture for me it is all fascinating.

I notice many people are very triggered by even the mere mention of Christianity. I get it - I have been that person myself. Often when people speak of Christianity, I find it's like we feel people are just telling us what to do. I think we have an innate mechanism built into us that for the most part we don't like to be bossed around or told what to do! On the other side of the coin, most of us also love a good story.

So for me I continue to stand by this as far as God is concerned: You may call it the Universal Life Force, the Creator, a power greater than yourself, or another name. Ultimately the Supreme

God of your understanding.

People from religious communities have also expressed fears that yoga is spiritually dangerous- I believe it is purely based in fear or a position of not knowing. When my dear mother once brought this concern up with me, I remember explaining succinctly, that I had come to a place of simply saying- No, to guilt and fear, and yes to greater consciousness and awareness.

Now that she is gone, I have had to go and revisit these ideas, and as a mother myself, address the religion of my upbringing. What do I really know about it? Usually if I opened the bible not much made sense or came at me in a negative way. It seemed at a glance, mixed up patriarchal and very cryptic. I continued to pray.

And I believe Jesus is *in* on this!

I believe in the idea of a loving God. A loving beyond brilliant creator. Beyond explanation, beyond comprehension, and that this consciousness truly does live within us. I also believe in a collective consciousness and a oneness we all share, and for me the teachings of Jesus Christ go right along with this. There is powerful healing in Christ consciousness, as long as you don't get too bogged down in the politics of it.

As I've gone along, I've opened myself to learning new things including about Christianity, God, the Bible and new things continue to be revealed to me. I continue to be drawn and called to the mystical, and the Bible definitely has its share of it.

Hatha Yoga

If you hear the word Hatha Yoga, it is referring to balance. Balancing the left and right, the sun and the moon, the hot and the cold, the inhale and the exhale. Yoga is the ancient and scientific side of joining the body, mind and spirit, and the sacred balance between the three.

The Mystical

In among my own personal explorations of the mystical, I have worked with Crystals and studied them and even created art based on them. All with the intentions of healing. To be perfectly honest, the original reason I was drawn to this is I wanted to create objects that would be able to heal all of our pain and troubles away. The idea was that these objects could be a conduit for healing - I felt deeply at the time there would be powerful value even by expressing the conceptual idea of it. I still believe in the power of crystals and gemstones, the colours of the rainbow and vibrations too. There is energy available to us in our natural environment. It might take practice, but it is something that can be noticed, felt out and worked with.

Prayer

Saying a prayer is a way of putting words to dreams, ideas and feelings. One thing I have truly found comfort and power in, in our times of distress, with the difficulties in our world is prayer. When there truly is not very much we can do, we can always pray. It is through prayer that I have learned, it is not always up to us to solve things. It's not always up to us to fix everything. Another thing I've found that goes along really well with prayer is listening.

Womens Spirituality - Sacred Cosmic Feminine.

As Far as the Sacred Feminine is concerned, I feel I must express that yes- no matter what- if you are a woman you are indelibly connected to this. Our own moon cycles, our bodies, our intuition, our womanhood is a source of great power and indeed an awesome thing to embrace.

As Women, considering our monthly cycle we are internally wired to resonate with ceremony and ritual.

It all relates to how we make sense and meaning of our lives. Most of us are not operating in this awareness very often, but with greater awareness can come greater meaning. People get fearful of it because it is so powerful to experience these connections. Yet as we face our fears - we shed light and bring deeper understanding.

Over 30 years ago. I picked up a book from a bookstore, It was titled, "A Woman's Book of Ritual" In smaller letters it was subtitled, "Casting the Circle". By Diane Stein. It was a long time ago and not really realizing what it entailed–I still remember being pleasantly surprised by what I read.

What I found in this book was an explanation of women's spirituality laid out in a friendly, readable manner. Simple and clear to understand, it was Wicca - and it said right at the beginning to remember whatever you send out with your intention comes back to you threefold, almost like the golden rule.

The writer explained the rituals and celebrations of cycles- the cycles of our lives, the cycles of the seasons and the cycles of the moon and she explained how it relates to women because of our menstrual cycles, and how it is special and powerful. Celebrating the seasons and moon cycles of the year, is connected to the earth and we are connected to the earth. I love the idea of women getting together and having these times of gathering, honouring life's passages and raising their energy and setting intentions towards creating the world we want to live in.

Alongside this I've studied the esoteric symbolism of tarot cards over the course of many years. I got my first tarot deck when I was about 12 years old. I can tell you I have found these cards can be a great tool for utilizing archetypal symbols to bring clarity and deeper meaning and awareness into the stories of our lives.

Another interesting book to mention in relation to this is Jean Shinoda Bolen's book Goddesses in All Women, which really explains archetypes in a very interesting way that you can understand and have fun with too.

Over the years I have met women who practice forms of wicca, and am honored to have participated in medicine circles that incorporate indigenous spirituality. I've learned through my own experience about the powerful, sometimes slippery magic of setting intentions, and visualization. I have felt the awesome cleansing power of burning earthy herbs, like sage and sweetgrass. As I continue to learn more about energy medicine, I truly more than ever recognise the connection between mother earth and God above and how none of it is separate, but very much interconnected, and how our spiritual energetic core is exactly what connects us to each other, the earth and to the heavens.

I recognize the conditioning. How religion has been used to control people, and hurt people too. I understand the terrible violence towards women and people in general over history, and the deeply ingrained fear it has instilled. I strongly empathize and honor and stand with all who agree with the need for healing to take place.

Non Violence

Ahimsa Is the Yoga Sanskrit Word for non-Violence- It is the number 1 of the first limb of the eight limbs of Yoga, To practice non-violence. It just seems such a simple concept, and yet the wars that seem to rise up even within our own selves can be so powerful, let alone, disagreements within families and between close friends. The Fears inside us, can lead to strong reactions, of fear, and anger and can then lead unchecked to...well violence - plain and simple. This even includes the destructive force of feeling mean towards yourself and beating yourself up. Finding ways to break down the walls of fear, and misunderstanding and learning how to make peace with yourself, take what is yours, find ways to deal with it and let go of the rest is on the path to non-violence. Yoga leads to meditation which leads to awareness, which leads to non-violence.

Staying Present- Meditation

Also being willing to stay with the present moment and whatever it is. Wow, this is powerful and challenging. Pema Chodron, the famous female Buddhist author, in her book "The Places that Scare You- A Guide to Fearlessness in Difficult Times"said, when faced with our own inner demons, most of us want to run screaming out of the room! But s that is the meditative practice- *To Stay*- To observe and to discover the humanity we share- to find the bodhicitta (aka our soft feeling heart and the path to enlightenment).

When we stay with the actual feeling it can move through and dissipate, this is true liberation, it's not as easy as it sounds, but all it takes is staying power.

Chakra Systems- Crystal Healing

The Chakra Systems of ancient India have always held great fascination for me. Colors, crystals, messages, signs, and symbols are all powerful, interesting and can bring us closer to enlightenment, and health. These are good things. These things can hold great information and tell us about ourselves. I know they have for me, but it's taken time and been quite a journey!

One art piece I built was a copper bodice with stone settings based on connections to the Chakra systems of the body. I did this with the intention of exploring the healing power of gemstones to heal us and even heal the world! I put quite a lot of energy into these activities and it was a privilege to be able to do it at an academic level. Although admittedly it was a great challenge learning the skills it took for this project; once I got to that point, it was also exciting, fun and rewarding.

Before I proceeded on this project I had to explore, I had to do research, and investigate my own ideas around it all.

I had to admit to myself when I began that at the time - besides my fascination with the idea, I didn't automatically see these energy centers in our bodies. But I asked myself, what if I looked inside? I clearly remember, consciously going to sit down outside under a tree, on the college campus. I closed my eyes and relaxed. Then I looked inside my body to see what I saw in the areas described to me in the various books I'd been reading, and low and behold the colors were actually there! From the base of the spine, to the top of the head is a progression of the rainbow, from dark red, to orange, to yellow to green to blue all the way up to purple and white.

What I've found out about all of this mystical stuff is- sure it is, it can be used as tools. I have also found focusing on and giving too much attention to these things can become in one word- obsessive. Anything taken too far, can take the joy out of it. With crystals, remember that if you think a stone is pretty or you like it, that is enough to tell you it is good for you. For me the goal is clarity, and anything in extremes takes things out of their balanced state. I love to deepen my understanding and awareness, for instance finding out that different crystals have different healing properties. At the same time, I like to practice allowing space for myself and others to be exactly where we are. Where we are is where it's at.

A note on energy- Since I've been writing this book my path has led me to learn and gather more information about energy awareness, energy medicine, and Reiki. I am learning more about things like our energetic core and how it relates to our connection between heaven and earth. As my awareness deepens and I see many connections yoga has to other healing modalities like acupressure, traditional chinese medicine meridians, Qi Gong, the chakras systems and our aura. The mystery continues to unfold. Who knows maybe the notes on energy will become another book? Time will tell.

Belief In A Higher Power

That Higher Power is inside us, we can hold space for it. We can as I like to say "Simplify Life to Live" . We can choose kindness, we can choose compassion, towards ourselves and others. We can remember that it is not all up to us. We are human, we don't have to know all the answers. As much as we would like to have certainty- The only thing that is certain is change. Letting our higher power lead can take a lot of pressure off of us.

I have found, when you take everything else away, there is a prevailing energy in our universe.

All we really need- is to stay present to it. But this is often a lot easier said than done. It's a beautiful thing that can vary greatly in intensity. Staying present means not only enjoying the moment for what it is, but also allowing ourselves to notice everything about it. This includes the many ways we either pull back, hide, and avoid experiences, or when and what we run towards. And all the things we use to soothe hurt or for protection from hurting that may actually numb us from our good feelings too, and keep us from living the true fullness of our life. Remembering to be gentle and loving towards our most vulnerable selves, when we can stay present we can find the golden nuggets of being alive!

Staying present is the key that moves the pain through and is a skill that has not often been taught. You are allowed to have your feelings, and your feelings are allowed to move and change. In fact, having mixed feelings according to Canadian psychologist Gordon Neufeld, is actually a sign of maturity! So there you have it.

From my own experience, I would say: Stay curious. When you feel fear -investigate. Try not to take yourself too seriously or at least begin to notice when you are. Also Sleep. I am learning a bit late in the game how important sleeping is. I'm by nature a bit of a night owl and I know that's ok, but sleep is maintenance medicine for the brain and body. Do whatever you can as a great act of kindness to yourself, in honour of your life, the world and your dreams - to wind down each day and get enough rest!

I decided to give Christianity a chance because it was the religion of my upbringing. I have struggled with it, and I have personally also found comfort.

Yes, there is oppression and yes there is conditioning, and then what? Then I believe there is still God.

I recognize my faults, and understand I am often more of a hopeless sinner than a mother Teresa. But no matter what I have found I can turn to God. God is there for me, and God is inside of me. This is what Christians mean by "The Good News" (Insert Big Smiley face) It also is part of recognizing the divine within and choosing to honor continuous unfoldment in ourselves within this amazing universe we live in.

Whatever it is you believe I honor you, and accept we don't have to believe the same things in the same way.!

But when it comes down to it, I have to be honest in my hours of need and always, -along with yoga and the healing energy tools I've gained- I personally rely on God.

The Lord is my Shepherd. Psalm 23

I find the hardest times in my life have been when I have lost sight of this so I just have to say it- and speak honestly here, as an expression of personal truth- praise the Lord, I believe in God.

…And I believe in rainbows too.

I realize our beliefs are personal and private, I am sharing here in part as a personal exercise in recognizing some of my beliefs, and finding how they actually contain many layers. I do not pass any judgment on anyone else, for anything. I feel deeply, it is not my place to judge. I respect other people's beliefs, and I hope that whoever reads this can find it in themselves to respect me for being honest about mine. Putting our beliefs into words can be challenging! As I've shared here formulating some words around those ideas we may carry around us you can be enlightening in itself.

May peace be with you & me & the universe- now and always.

Just Remember:

You get to be you, in your body in this life, and there is room for everyone! Life really is fascinating. People may from time to time judge or laugh at us. We can also laugh at ourselves, and people will laugh with us. People may steal from you, but they can also be very surprisingly generous, giving and forgiving. People may hurt you, and then people may hold space for you. Compassion starts with yourself, saying something accepting to yourself. People can be clever, funny and even when they are not, even when we are the complete opposite of clever and funny, we have lessons to teach each other, and although it's not always easy, in a way that is clever and funny in itself.

The trick is not to allow anything to stop us from going forward with our lives. Keep your eye on your north start, head towards your greatest purposes. And if you have stopped, just take a deep breath and step forward again, one baby step at a time. Keep breathing and observing all the flavors of life.

Certainly, sometimes we need to stop, have a rest and regroup, and then keep going.

Always continue to follow your dreams. Remember daydreaming is underrated !

In busy traffic, I have a habit of saying "Keep it flowing people!" I believe it applies here too.

When you are wounded how do you bounce back? How do you cope? What can you do to get back on your feet? How can you forgive yourself, others, the world, the failed expectations, the ego? What can you do? It's not always easy, it really isn't.

But are you breathing? Can you feel it? Can you hear it? Can you stop the judgements and notice it ? This is Yoga. This is the present moment, and it is all we ever really have.

CONCLUSION

It is with much gratitude that I offer my sincere Thanks for reading along.

My hope is you may continue to find ways of feeling truly well from the inside and out on all levels- physical, mental, and spiritual. That you may find peace and comfort in the poses and ideas here and incorporate them into your own personal daily health routine. More often than not through kindness & acceptance of exactly where you are at in the present moment. You've got this!

Final reminders to remember : Go slowly, be easy on yourself. Remember this is surprisingly not about achieving any outcome! It is about giving yourself a little space to be you in your body. Honestly, the slower the better! Give yourself the chance to explore exactly what is going on inside you, it's an amazing thing.

The yoga poses I have presented are a framework to help this to happen. Notice your breathing. Always go back to the breath and check in. Can you take 5 conscious breaths? This is the beginning, and allow yourself the freedom of being a beginner. The breath is the connection between the body and the mind. The Breath is the key.

Through a little bit of yoga practice you can find a path to wellness that works for you. May we all find peace in the true authentic in and out flow of the moment and simplify our lives to live.

The biggest reason I wrote this little Yoga book is to share with you the opportunity to put yourself into these yoga poses and actually give yourself a chance to experience the life affirming aspects of Yoga.

Much Love,

Holly Kirkpatrick Ulrich 2022

ACKNOWLEDGEMENT

Many thanks and blessings go out to all who have been there along my life's pathway.

First to my husband Joe and my son Nolan, the sweetest loves of my life. Thank you both for your love and patience ,
supporting my efforts to write this book. You deserve hugs and kisses and milk chocolate with nuts!

My dear family and friends near and far who continue to show up, in big and small ways – please know you are in my heart. I love and appreciate you very much.

With Gratitude and reverence to my Yoga Teachers:

Rockne White - Thank you for creating Yoga in Motion, now known as Yoga Passage, at just the right moment for me to walk in and be your first customer! Thank you for your great enthusiasm, generosity, and support. I have learned so much from you and am grateful for our enduring friendship.
Val Petrich - Thank you for including me, for the teachings at yoga studio college, and for believing in me, when I didn't even know I needed it. I really enjoyed working for you.
Kathy Nash- My first yoga teacher. Thank you for lifting me up off the ground and lighting the spark with your teachings.

Also Thanks to a few more favourites: David Williams for sharing your experiential knowledge of advanced ashtanga vinyasa yoga. Daniel Pechie for being so effective in inspiring embodied esoteric wisdom. Judith Hansen Lasater for sharing the delicious restorative aspects of yoga. Larry Schultz, for making yoga cool. And so many more amazing people who I have crossed paths with in the yoga world.

I am blessed to have met you - and it's been so much fun! You are all true universal stars.

Finally, I would like to give thanks to all the people who were my people at some point, and always will be in the time space continuum, because love is like water - It does not quit flowing.

From the bottom of my heart-
Huge Loving Gratitude and Hugs always,

Holly Kirkpatrick Ulrich

2022

ABOUT THE AUTHOR

Holly Kirkpatrick Ulrich

Holly is a writer, dreamer, artist and life lover. She is from the far Northern Interior of British Columbia Canada. She did her yoga training in Calgary Canada. She wrote this book while living in the Swiss Alps, with her dear husband and darling son.

You can find out more about her work through her website: www.evamarieoriginals.com

"YOGA LIFESAVERS, MY YOGA STORY HANDBOOK"

By Holly Kirkpatrick Ulrich
Memorial Street 1,
Muotathal, Schwyz
Switzerland

evamarieoriginal@gmail.com

Eva Marie Originals

www.evamarieoriginals.com